PROSTATE CANCER

Awareness Booklet

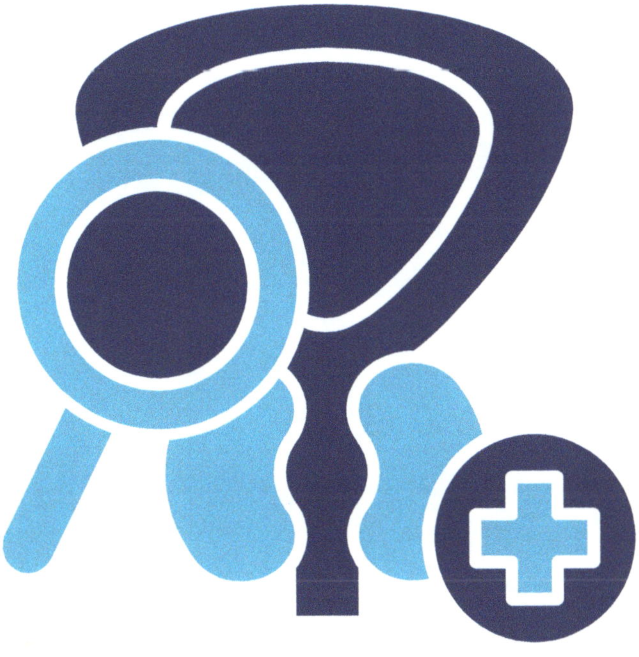

Together,
Let's raise awareness and support the ongoing fight against prostate cancer because every voice and action counts.

By Delatria Sam

Prostate Cancer Awareness Booklet: For the ones who walk with quiet strength

ISBN: 979-8-3496-2410-0

Dedication

To those who have fought, those who are fighting, and those who will face Prostate Cancer, may this booklet provide knowledge, hope, and strength.

What is Prostate Cancer?

It is a type of cancer that occurs in the prostate gland, a small gland in the male reproductive system.

Common Symptoms:

- Difficulty urinating
- Frequent urination
- Blood in urine or semen
- Painful urination or ejaculation

Treatment Options:

- Vary depending on the stage and aggressiveness of the cancer, ranging from active surveillance to surgery
- Radiation
- Hormone therapy

Awareness and regular check-ups are crucial for early detection and effective management.

In the following 10 pages, you'll read inspiring stories from individuals who have been impacted by prostate cancer. These personal accounts share experiences, challenges, and triumphs from patients, caregivers, fighters, supporters, and healers. Their stories highlight the importance of awareness, support, and resilience in the face of prostate cancer. We hope these stories inspire and motivate you to take action, whether it's getting screened, supporting a loved one, or advocating for prostate cancer awareness.

John’s Second Chance: My Doctor's Words Changed Everything

“I was diagnosed with prostate cancer at 60. My doctor's calm and reassuring words made all the difference. Treatment went smoothly, and I'm grateful for that second chance.”

Mark’s Faith Journey: Finding Strength in Faith

“When I was diagnosed with advanced prostate cancer, my faith helped me cope. I'm focusing on my health and cherishing time with loved ones.”

Supporting My Husband: Sarah's Support

"When my husband was diagnosed, I felt lost. But I became his rock, driving him to appointments and managing his care. We're facing this together."

Maria: A Mother's Support

“My son's diagnosis affected our whole family. I'm proud of how we've rallied around him, offering love and support every step of the way.”

I’m Not Alone! David’s Support System

“I've met incredible men through support groups who understand what I'm going through. We're in this fight together.”

Living With Purpose: Alex's New Purpose

"After treatment, I realized life is precious. Now, I focus on helping others and spreading awareness about prostate cancer."

A Friend's Support: Emily's Friend in Need

"When my friend was diagnosed, I wanted to help. We talk regularly, and I've learned so much about prostate cancer."

My Father's Legacy: James' Legacy

“Losing my father to prostate cancer motivated me to spread awareness. “

Compassionate Care: Nurse Rachel's Compassion

"As a nurse, I strive to provide emotional support and educate patients about their options. It's rewarding to see patients thrive."

Advancing Treatment: Dr Patel's Breakthrough

"As a researcher, I'm working to develop more effective treatments. Every breakthrough brings us closer to beating prostate cancer."

SELF-CARE

EVEN ON TOUGH DAYS

Take a relaxing bath after treatment

Listen to calming music during check-ups

Write in a Prostate Cancer journal

Spend time outdoors for a mood boost

Do gentle exercises for prostate health

Enjoy a warm beverage for comfort

Treat yourself to a favorite healthy snack

Watch an uplifting movie during recovery

Reach out to a Prostate Cancer support friend

RESEARCH UPDATE

Researchers are exploring combination therapies and immunotherapy in clinical trials.

PATIENT RIGHTS AND RESPONSIBILITIES

YOUR RIGHTS

You will be treated with dignity and respect, safely and humanely, regarding your prostate cancer diagnosis and treatment.

We respect your religious, ethnic, and personal values in the context of prostate cancer care.

You will receive education on how to manage your prostate cancer care at home.

Protecting the privacy and confidentiality of your prostate cancer-related information is a top priority.

You are entitled to know the names of healthcare professionals responsible for your prostate cancer care.

YOUR RESPONSIBILITIES

Describe your medical history in detail, including any history of prostate issues or family history of prostate cancer.

Let us know if any problems arise or if your medical condition related to prostate cancer changes.

Be respectful to our staff, patients, and visitors during your prostate cancer treatment.

Comply with the hospital regulations regarding prostate cancer treatment and care.

Payments for medical services related to prostate cancer must be made on time.

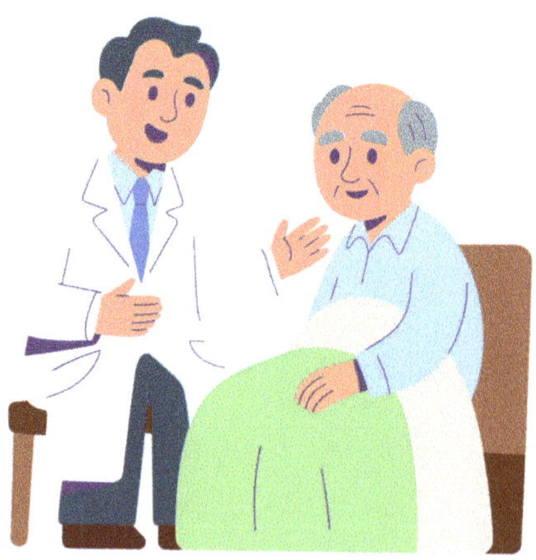

Did You *Know?*

Prostate cancer often grows slowly, and early detection can significantly improve treatment outcomes.

4 WAYS TO RAISE PROSTATE CANCER AWARENESS

Spread the Facts

Be There for Patients

Make Some Noise

Get Involved in Events

Did You *Know?*

Prostate cancer screening typically involves: (1) Digital Rectal Exam (DRE): A doctor feels the prostate gland for abnormalities. (2) Prostate-Specific Antigen (PSA): A blood test measures PSA levels; it can be elevated in men with prostate cancer.

HAVE YOU BEEN SCREENED?

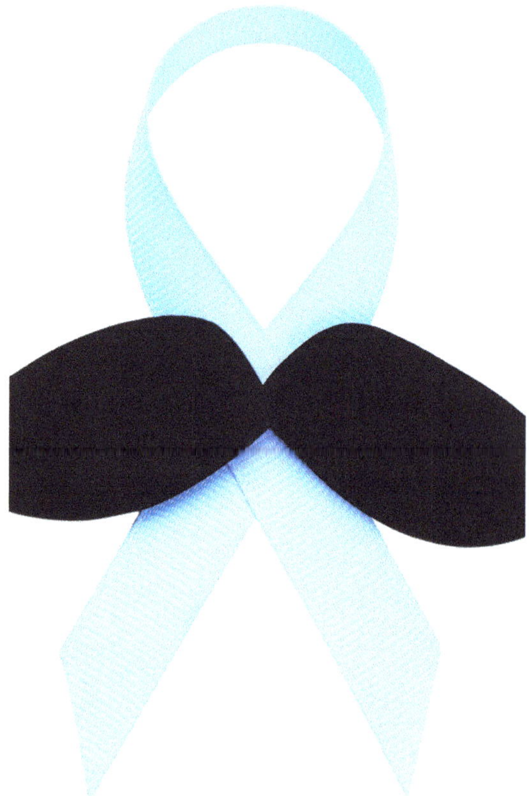

SEPTEMBER IS

PROSTATE CANCER

AWARENESS MONTH

Don't wait! Talk to your doctor about getting screened for prostate cancer. Early detection saves lives.

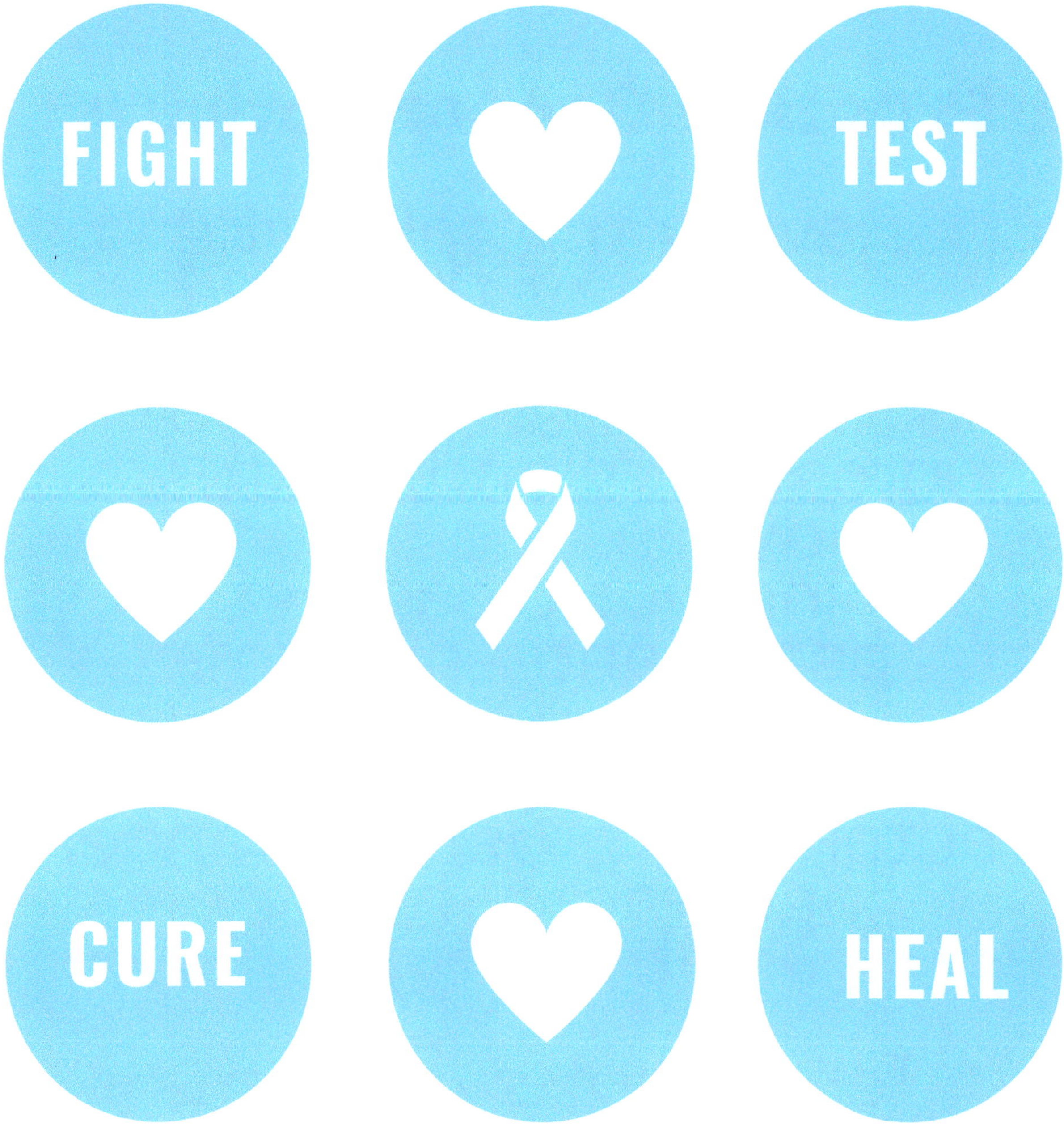

LET'S BE AWARE

We can fight Prostate Cancer together

LEARN THE SYMPTOMS AND
GET A CHECK-UP TODAY!

VISIT
PROSTATECANCER.ORG
FOR MORE INFORMATION

Prostate Cancer Activity

Review the following diagram of the male reproductive system, studying parts like the prostate gland, testes, epididymis, vas deferens, seminal vesicles, urethra, penis, and scrotum.

Grab a friend, discuss risk factors for prostate cancer (age, family history, ethnicity).

Talk about symptoms (difficulty urinating, weak urine flow, etc) and the importance of screenings like PSA tests.

Understanding the Male Reproductive System

To educate about the male reproductive system, focusing on the prostate gland and its relation to prostate cancer.

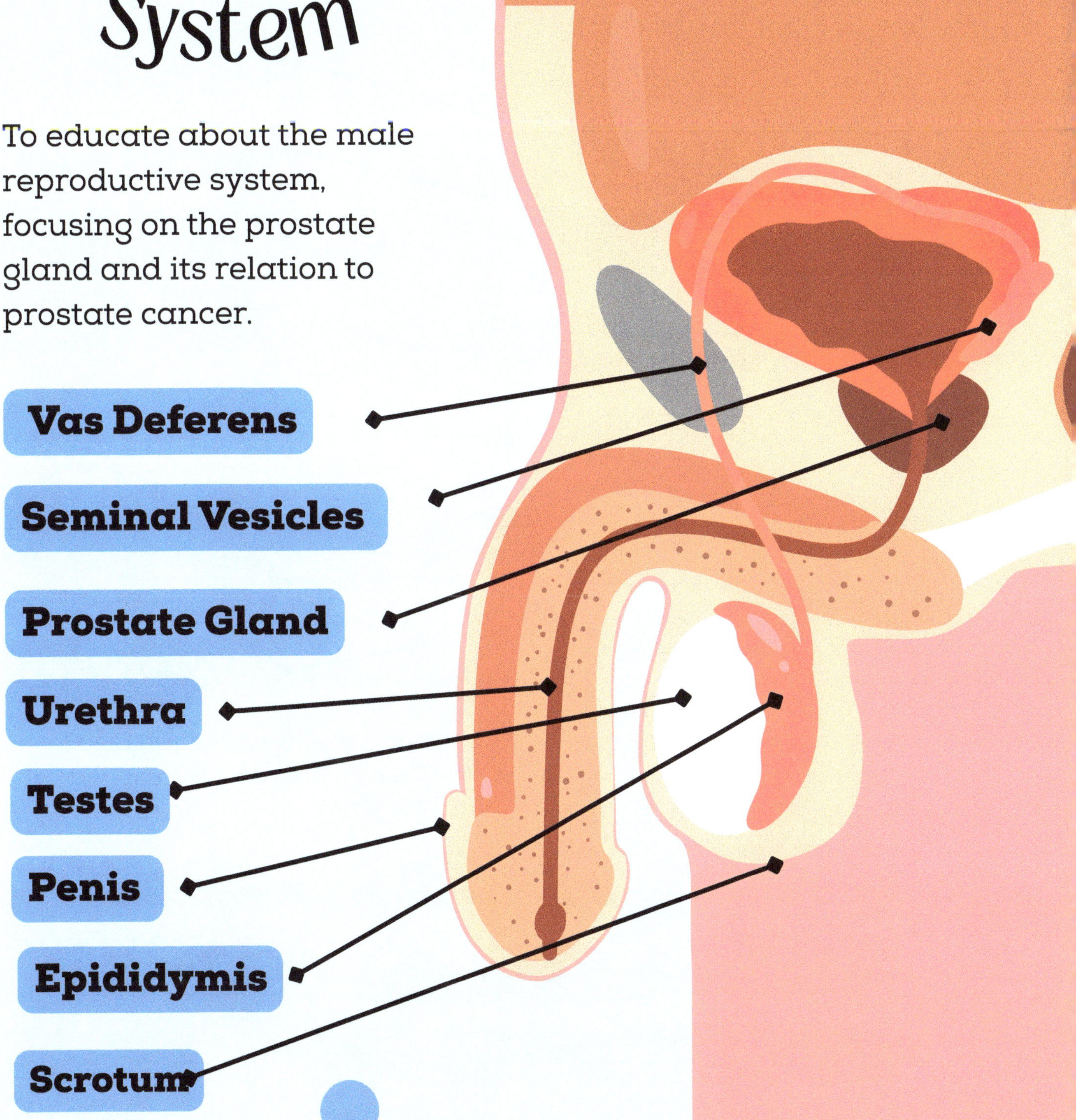

Now it's your turn!

Can you identify the parts of the Male Reproductive System?

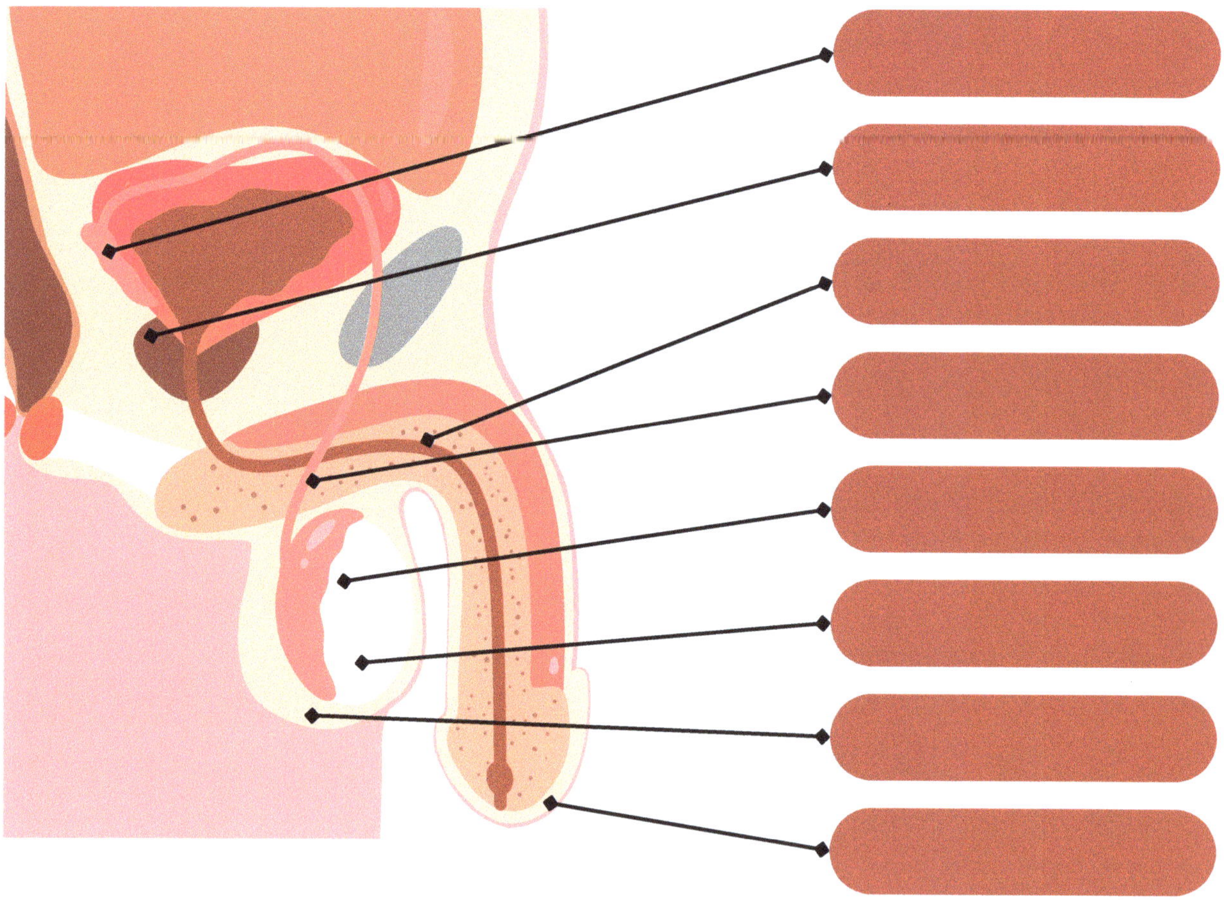

Write the names of each part of the male reproductive system in their respective locations as indicated by the lines pointing to different parts of the diagram.

Penis	**Vas Deferens**	**Urethra**
Epididymis	**Seminal Vesicles**	**Testes**
Scrotum	**Prostate Gland**	

Let's discuss how the Male Reproductive System Works!

Reproductive System

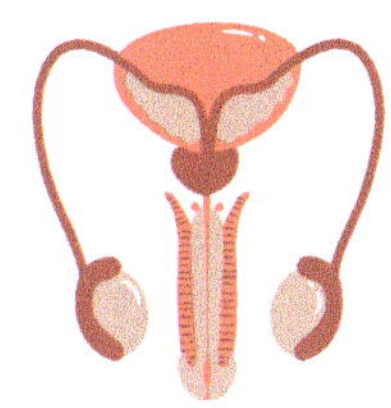

Penis	The penis is involved in urination and the delivery of sperm during ejaculation.
Epididymis	The epididymis stores and matures sperm from the testes before they move to the vas deferens.
Scrotum	The scrotum is a sac of skin that houses and protects the testes, regulating their temperature for sperm development.
Vas Deferens	The vas deferens transports sperm from the epididymis to the urethra in preparation for ejaculation.
Seminal Vesicles	Seminal vesicles produce a significant portion of the fluid that makes up semen, providing nutrients for sperm.
Prostate Gland	The prostate gland produces additional fluid for semen and helps control urination.
Urethra	The urethra is a tube that carries both urine and semen out of the body.
Testes	The testes produce sperm and testosterone, a hormone crucial for male development and reproductive function

Writing Facts!
Prostate Cancer

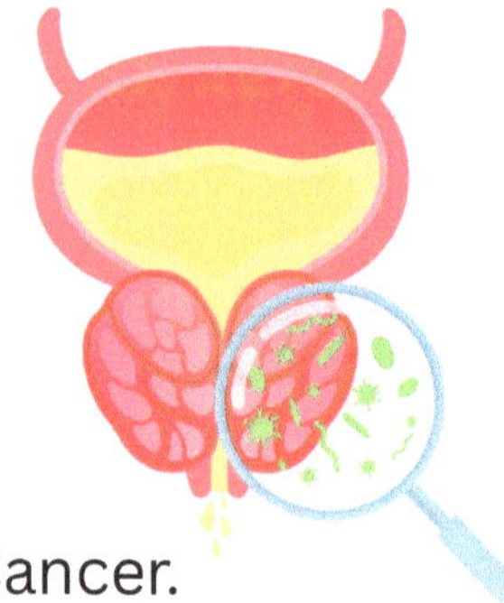

Write some fun facts you learned about Prostate Cancer.

Let's talk Prostate Health!

Here are 4 ways to keep your Prostate healthy.

Regular Screening: Get regular check-ups and screenings for prostate health, like PSA (Prostate-Specific Antigen) tests, especially after age 50	**Healthy Diet**: Eat a diet rich in fruits, vegetables, and foods high in lycopene (such as tomatoes), which may help support prostate health.
Stay Active: Exercise regularly to maintain overall health and potentially reduce risks associated with prostate issues.	**Don't Smoke:** Avoid smoking, as it can increase risks for various health problems, including potentially impacting overall reproductive and prostate health.

NOW LET'S TEST YOUR KNOWLEDGE

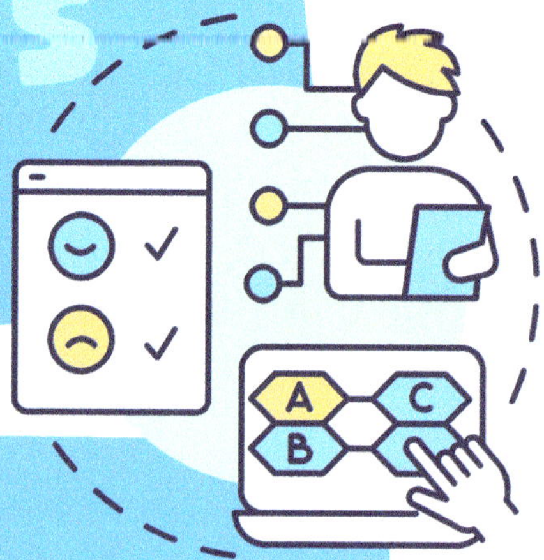

Q: What is the function of the prostate gland in the male reproductive system?

A:

Q: Which part of the male reproductive system produces sperm?

A:

Q: What is one common cancer affecting the male reproductive system?

A:

MAKE A LIST!

What do you want to know about prostate cancer? Make a list of questions or topics you'd like to learn more about regarding prostate cancer, symptoms, screenings, or support.

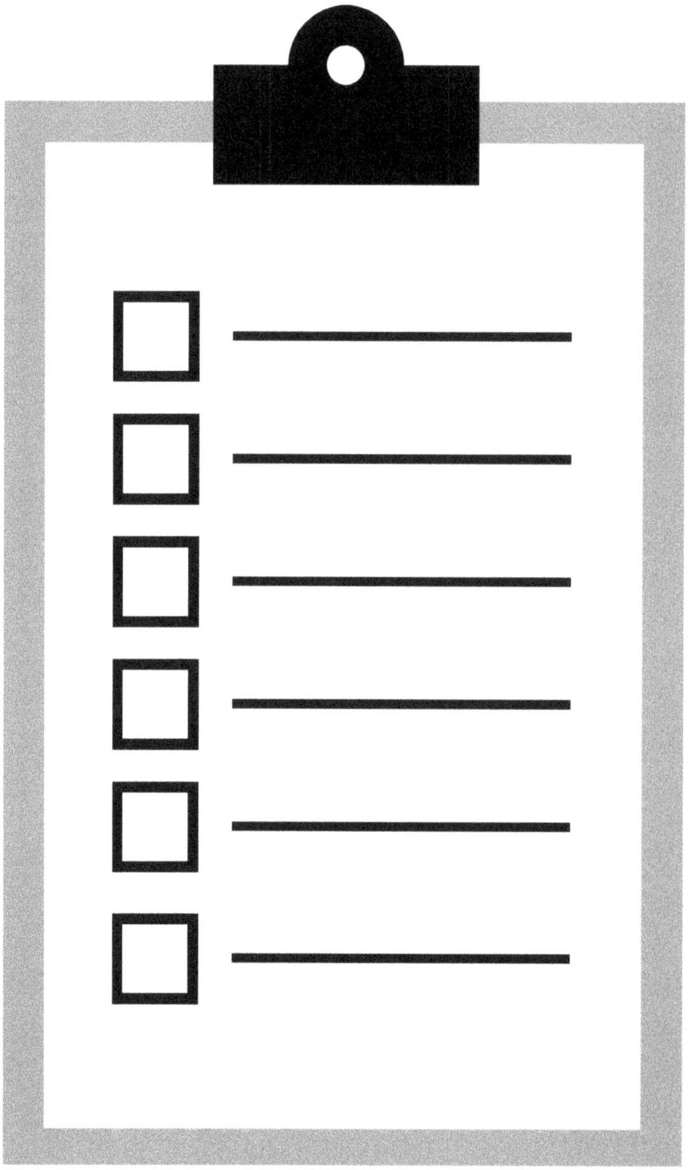

LET'S PACK!

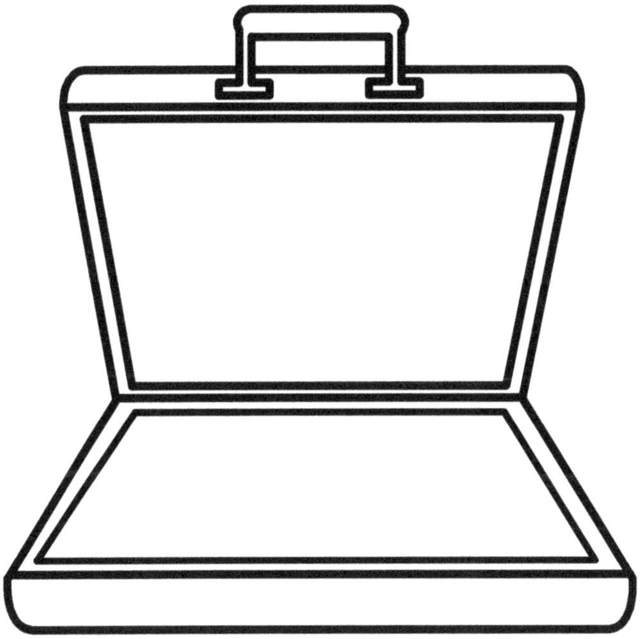

What would you like to include in your Prostate Cancer bag? Draw pictures of things that symbolize support, awareness, or resources for prostate cancer.

Did You *Know?*

Some foods thought to support prostate health include: Tomatoes, Green Tea, and Broccoli.

TIME TO EAT!

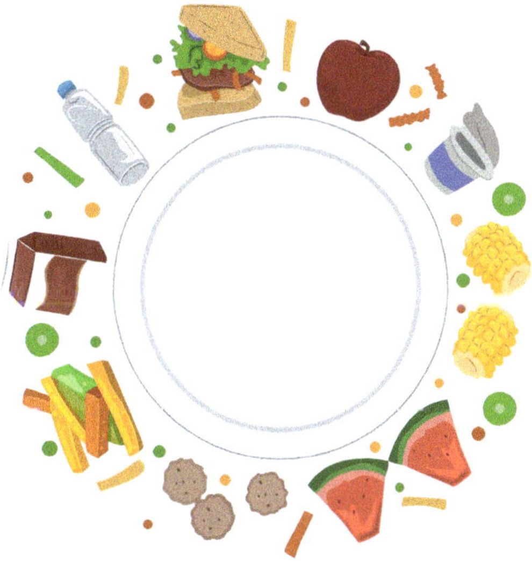

Name the top 3 foods that are nutritious for prostate health. Write their names and your opinions about them.

1-

2-

3-

GET SOCIAL!

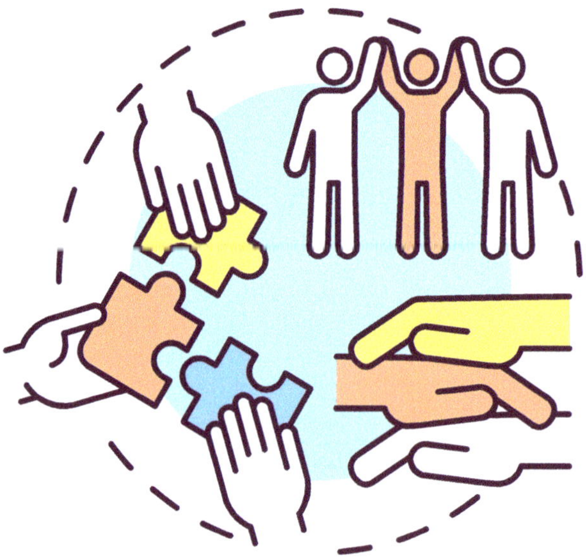

Meet 3 new people who are involved in or care about prostate cancer awareness. Learn a fact about each person related to awareness, research, support, or prevention.. Write those facts down in the space below.

GRAB YOUR DIARY!

Choose the best day of your involvement in Prostate Cancer Awareness. Write what happened in your diary about how you supported, learned about, or spread awareness on prostate cancer.

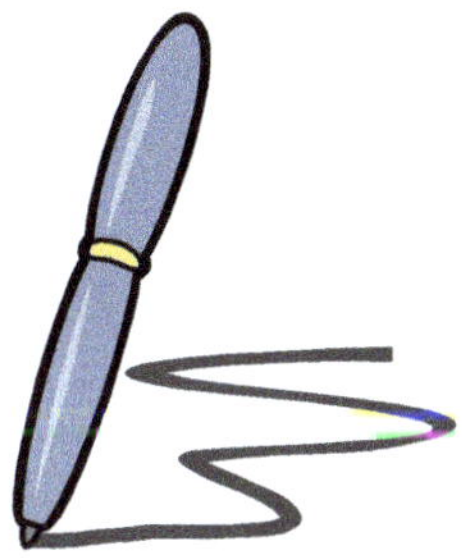

LISTEN!

What do you hear about prostate cancer awareness? Listen to the conversations around you or thoughts in your mind about Prostate Cancer. Draw pictures or write down messages you hear related to prostate cancer awareness.

DON'T FORGET READING!

Read a book about prostate cancer. Write its title, genre, author, and illustrator. You can note down 3 new words you've learned from the book.

The importance of

REGULAR HEALTH CHECK-UPS

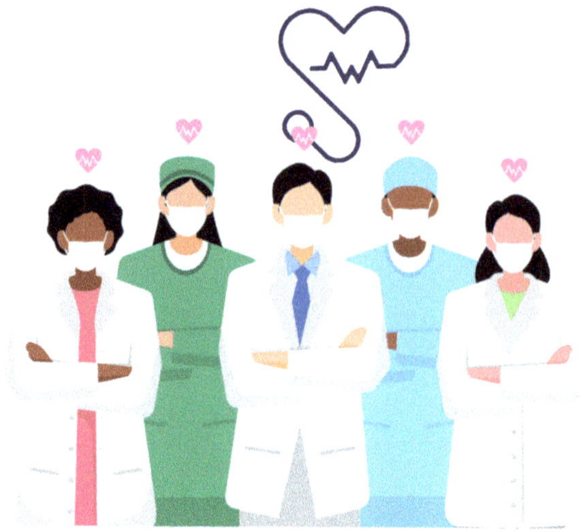

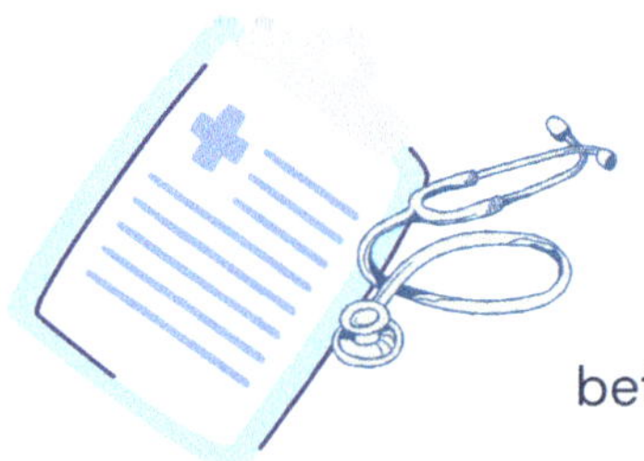

Early Detection of Health Issues

Regular check-ups can lead to early detection of prostate cancer, potentially before symptoms appear—early detection is key for effective treatment and better outcomes.

Promotion of Healthy Lifestyle

A healthy lifestyle can contribute to overall health and potentially reduce risks associated with various cancers, including prostate cancer. Healthcare professionals can offer guidance during check-ups.e

The importance of regular health check-ups

Preventive Care

Health check-ups include screenings and assessments that can identify risk factors for prostate cancer. Screenings like PSA (Prostate-Specific Antigen) tests are part of the preventive care for men at risk.

Monitoring Chronic Conditions

For men with chronic conditions or at higher risk for prostate cancer, regular monitoring is vital for managing health and making informed decisions about care.

– MEDICAL GLOSSARY –

PROSTATE CANCER ESSENTIALS

TERM	MEDICAL MEANING
Prostate	A gland in the male reproductive system.
Prostate Cancer	Cancer that forms in the prostate gland.
PSA (Prostate-Specific Antigen)	A protein made by the prostate, used in screenings.
Screening	Tests to detect cancer before symptoms appear.
Biopsy	Removing tissue to check for cancer cells.
Diagnosis	Determining the presence of cancer.

– MEDICAL GLOSSARY –

PROSTATE CANCER ESSENTIALS

TERM	MEDICAL MEANING
Treatment	Methods to manage or cure prostate cancer.
Risk Factors	Things that increase prostate cancer likelihood.
Symptoms	Signs that might indicate prostate cancer.
Early Detection	Finding cancer early for better outcomes.
Active Surveillance	Monitoring slow-growing prostate cancer.
Prognosis	Outlook for recovery or disease progression.

TESTIMONIAL

"I thought I was invincible, but prostate cancer had other plans. Early detection saved my life. Now, I'm passionate about spreading awareness and encouraging men to get screened."

John, Survivor

TESTIMONIAL

TESTIMONIAL
TESTIMONIAL

"Losing my dad to prostate cancer was devastating. But I'm determined to honor his memory by fighting for more research and better care for those affected."

Emily, Caregiver

TESTIMONIAL

TESTIMONIAL

TESTIMONIAL

"As a doctor, I've seen firsthand how prostate cancer can impact lives. But with advancements in treatment and early detection, I'm optimistic about the future for those diagnosed."

Dr. Smith, Oncologist

In loving

MEMORY OF ALL

Those We Lost to Prostate Cancer

A TRIBUTE TO THE LIVES TOUCHED BY PROSTATE CANCER, HONORING THE MEMORY OF LOVED ONES WHO BATTLED THIS DISEASE.

www.ingramcontent.com/pod-product-compliance
Lightning Source LLC
LaVergne TN
LVHW070858210926
848482LV00016B/970